I0439763

Facial Exercises

Remove Wrinkles & Enjoy A Younger Looking Face with Face Yoga

Table of Contents

Introduction

Did you know that each person has a different number of facial muscles? That is strange, right? Are you also aware that you can get rid of wrinkles and look younger by simply doing facial exercises? Cool isn't it. Most people exercise various body muscles and forget the facial muscles that also need to be exercised in order to look healthier and younger.

Are you looking to look ten years younger? Do you want to get rid of those annoying wrinkles? Are you tired of having to get Botox injections frequently in order to have that younger looking skin? Then you are in the right place because Face yoga is the natural alternative to Botox, face lifts and over the counter anti-aging creams – minus the harmful consequences of course! But what exactly is face yoga and what does I do?

The Reasoning Behind Face Yoga

In order to understand how exactly face yoga works, you need to keep in mind the two main functions of facial muscles. Facial muscles:

Enable you to express emotions

As a human being, you experience different emotions each day. Your facial muscles allow you to show the emotions you are experiencing without putting those emotions in words. You can express pain, happiness, surprise, sadness and other emotions by the use of just your facial muscles.

Shape your face

Facial muscles are not thinly spread out. They come in layers and they form around the cranium and facial tissues. As they form, your face begins taking shape. This is why the face can be categorized into different shapes.

These two functions of facial muscles, as beneficial as they are, also bring about wrinkles, drooping eyelids, laugh lines, and double chins (sagging neckline). For instance, your facial muscles enable you to show emotions. For example, they enable you to frown and express laughter. However, as you continue laughing or frowning, you are also putting tension on the muscles around your nose and mouth. This tension, over a period, leads to sagging lines. So, because you are putting tension on particular muscles, other areas near it begin to sag. When you laugh for instance, your cheeks become puffy, while the area around your nose and above your mouth sinks in. Thus, over some time, the tension stays on your cheeks while the other areas keep sagging.

This is where face yoga comes in to correct the situation.

Face yoga works in two ways. These are:

It removes tension on your facial muscles

As you go about living your life, you rarely think of the facial expressions you make. You may once in awhile, point to someone else as you notice his or her facial expressions but this observation is rarely used on oneself. Face exercises work to release tension on the facial muscles you use. As we have already seen, this tension builds up to bring about sag lines and wrinkles. Once the tension is eliminated by use of facial exercises, your face starts to acquire that youthfulness it lost. However, just releasing tension is not enough. This brings us to the second part of face yoga.

It tones and tightens your facial muscles

Face yoga works to tone and firm up your facial muscles. Once you release the tension, you need to tone the muscles. This will lead to the tightening of the skin that had started to sag and prevent further drooping.

Face yoga uses fingers, as it is not possible to use things like weights to enhance toning of your face. In addition to toning your face, there are other benefits associated with facial exercises. Let us look at these in the next chapter.

Benefits of Face Yoga

So, what are some benefits of face yoga?

You can do it on your own

Aging, busy lifestyles and the stress brought on by various situations, work to constantly beat you up and tear you down. You don't need to add to the list a stranger poking around on your face or marking problem areas that need some work. You can easily do facial exercises in your home and away from prying eyes. In addition, you don't need a lot of strength or any equipment in order to perform face yoga. All you need are your fingers. That alone is a worthwhile benefit to engage in face yoga.

You don't have to break the bank

The thing with Botox and facial creams is that they cost money. You could consider it an investment if it was a one off fee but you constantly have to replenish your supply and get new injections and before you know it, you have spent a fortune on solutions that don't last. On the other hand, facial exercises do not require cash. All you need to do is spend a few minutes to exercise your face muscles and the benefits make it time well spent.

You don't have to worry about toxins

Every other day on news sites and blogs, there are stories of surgeries gone wrong or photos of people who ended up looking like something out of a horror movie because of Botox injections gone wrong or due to allergic reactions because of using some facial creams. It's no wonder that most creams come with a warning to stop using them if you notice an allergic reaction. However, you don't have to worry about negative effects and allergic reactions when it comes to doing facial exercises. They are non-toxic.

Face Yoga keeps your face stress-free

When you are stressed, your muscles bear the brunt of the tension. It's not unusual for people to say that someone 'looks stressed' – it shows on your face and it also builds up on your chin, jaw and neck muscles. Engaging in facial exercises eliminates the stress from these areas and helps you feel relaxed.

Face Yoga helps you build confidence

Face yoga acts to stimulate the production of collagen. This in turn keeps your face looking healthy and youthful. When you look good, your outlook on life changes simply because you have added confidence. You don't have to worry about how others perceive you and you go about living your life to the fullest.

Face Yoga does not rob you of your humanity

One thing that surgery often does is rob people of their humanity. Human beings are feeling beings. They tend to express such feelings through words and the use of facial muscles. Surgery and Botox tend to keep the muscles in a permanent freeze. Once you get the injections, you are unable to convey your expressions. You acquire that 'plastic look' that is far removed from humanity. Face yoga removes tension without robbing you of the ability to express your emotions.

Yes, there are many benefits associated with doing facial exercises. However, knowing about face yoga or the benefits it comes with is just the first step in getting rid of wrinkles and reclaiming your youthful appearance. The next step is learning and actually doing the facial exercises. However, before engaging in facial exercises, it is important to prepare adequately.

How to Prepare for Face Yoga

Face yoga, like any other exercise, needs some forethought. Keep in mind that you will be training muscles. Some of these muscles have not been used for some time; hence the need to do certain things in order to ease into doing the yoga. You should:

Schedule face yoga time

Do not leave facial exercises to chance. If you do, you will be less inclined to do them. You need to schedule a specific time to engage in face yoga. You can set aside two days in a week to do facial exercises. Schedule a start date and stick to it. The time you schedule should be convenient for you. During this time, you should be able to finish the exercise routine without disruptions. Disruptions break the exercise routine and that is not good when exercising as you will not reap the full benefits of face yoga. If you can include face yoga in your morning routine, it is advisable to do so. This way, doing facial exercises will gradually become a normal part of a familiar routine.

Clean your hands

Your hands are your 'gym equipment' when it comes to face yoga. Unfortunately, hands carry germs with them. You do not want germs transferred to your face, as this will lead to another set of problems altogether. Pimples and whiteheads thrive on skin as bacteria takes root. Keep bacteria away from your face by thoroughly washing your hands before you begin.

Cleanse your face

After you have washed your hands, you need to wash your face. This is why it's advisable to add face yoga as part of your bathing routine. Your face is delicate. The skin on your face is thinner than that of other parts of the body. You have to be gentle yet thorough when washing your face. You can apply moisturizer after you are done to keep your skin moist. The moisturizer you use will depend on your skin type.

Once you are done with face yoga preparation, it is time to start the actual facial exercises. You can do various exercises but as you start out, you may want to concentrate on the areas that are starting to sag and wrinkle. You may also start from the top going down. Let us now look at the facial exercises you should engage in.

Facial Exercises

Forehead Exercise

Your forehead is very noticeable as far as your face goes. Unfortunately, it is also one of the facial parts that bear the brunt of wrinkles and sagging. Many people develop 'character lines' simply because they are so used to certain facial expressions that cause their forehead skin to fold. Worry is part of human life but it is also reflected on your forehead. Worry lines can become a permanent feature on your forehead (even when you are not worried). Keep in mind that tension tends to cause wrinkles and sagging. Therefore repeated actions, lead to undesirable effects. Forehead exercises will help you maintain a youthful appearance, as they will remove the tension on your forehead and allow the skin to go back to where it should have been.

There are three regions on the forehead: the upper, the mid and the lower region. Forehead exercises should take care of all these regions. In order to exercise your lower forehead, you should:

-Take your right index finger and place it above your right eyebrow in a horizontal position. Then take your left index finger and place it above your left eyebrow in a horizontal position. Ensure that both fingers flat on the skin.

-Once both your fingers are in place, gently pull down. You should feel your skin pulling down. In order to offer resistance, begin raising your eyebrows. This should work as added weight and help work the muscles.

-As you raise your eyebrows, remember to 'hold' for a moment before lowering them again and repeat the process at least fifteen times before stopping.

Once you are done with the lower forehead exercises, you need to move on. In order to work out the mid and upper area of your forehead, you should:

-Take your right hand and place four fingers near your right eyebrow in a vertical position such that your fingers lay on your temple. Ensure that the fingers are flat on your forehead. Then take your left hand and place four fingers near your left brow in a vertical position, making sure they are flat on your skin and touching the temple.

-After your left and right fingers are in place, gently stretch your forehead skin. Use your fingers to provide the needed stretch.

-Slowly begin to raise your eyebrows and then lower them. This will work in opposition to the stretching and provide resistance. Ensure that you repeat the exercise 15-20 times instead of doing it continuously.

-As you do your forehead exercises, you may feel a burning or pulling sensation. This is normal and it indicates you are on the right path. Once you are done with your forehead, you should move on to other parts of your face.

Between Eyebrows

The skin between your eyebrows is another area that wrinkles and sagging appears. When you worry or when you scowl, deep lines may appear. Your skin may look like a valley, with raised sides and a sunken center. As time goes by, the look may stay with you even when you are not scowling. You don't want to appear as the person who is always scowling even when you are not. Fortunately, you can use facial exercises to correct the situation. In order to exercise the facial muscles between your eyebrows, you should:

-Take your right hand and place four fingers above your right eyebrow in a horizontal position. Ensure that your fingers are flat on your forehead.

-Take your left hand and place four fingers above your left eyebrow ensuring that it is in a horizontal position.

-Once both hands are in place, begin pulling the skin away from the center and towards your temples. Your left hand should pull towards your left temple and vice versa.

-As you pull, scowl. That is, work to bring your eyebrows together. This will give your fingers some resistance to work against and ensure that your facial muscles get a good work out. If you feel a pulling or burning sensation, do not worry about it. Just continue with your exercises, stopping and starting again several times (at least ten times).

Upper Eyelids

Have you ever seen someone with droopy eyelids? Eyelids that seem to be closing although the person is wide awake. It is not a pretty sight. Unfortunately, as you continue to age, your eyelids begin to sag. This is especially true if you already have a sagging forehead because as your forehead sags, it also pushes down your eyelids. In order to correct the sagging, you need to work the upper eyelid muscles – muscles that make it possible for you to lift your eyelids. In order to exercise the muscle, you should:

-Take your right index finger and place it at the bottom of your right eyebrow in a horizontal position. Be careful not to poke your eye.

-Once your right finger is in position, gently lower your right eyebrow. Use your finger to provide resistance such that you have to struggle a bit to lower your eyebrow. Hold your finger in position, counting to five before releasing it. Repeat the exercises at least fifteen times.

-Once you are done with your right upper eyelid, take your left index finger and place it beneath your left eyebrow in a horizontal position.

-Use your left index finger to provide resistance as you lower your left eyebrow. Hold your left finger in position before releasing and repeat the exercise at least fifteen times.

You should be careful when exercising the muscles at the bottom of your eyebrow. Your eyes are delicate and should be handled with care. Once you are done with your upper eyelids, you should begin work on the lower part of your eye.

Lower Part of Eye Exercises

Various things can cause 'b-ags' to appear underneath your eyes. If you go to bed exhausted and wake up before your body is fully rested, you will end up with puffy bags underneath your eyes. Bags may also develop underneath your eyes when you retain excess fluid usually because of taking foods with a lot of salt. However, there are times when bags start to form due to the skin losing its elasticity.

Bags caused by the first two reasons tend to disappear after awhile. However, bags caused due to loss of elasticity become a permanent feature on your face. They make you look very tired and they 'increase' the years on your face. This situation only worsens with the passage of time. No one wants to have drooping bags underneath their eyes. It is not an inviting sight. In order to correct the situation, you should:

-Take your right index finger and place it at the bottom of the drooping lower eyelid. The finger should be at par with the middle of your nose. It should not be on top of the drooping part.

-Once your finger is in place, pull gently. Your eye is delicate and you don't want to injure it just to exercise its muscles. As you pull gently, try closing your eye. This will work to create resistance as your finger will be working to pull away as the action of shutting your eye will be working against your finger. Do not shut your eye all the way.

-Hold your finger in position by counting to five before releasing. Begin the exercise again until you have done it at least ten times.

-Once you are done with your right eye, switch to the left eye. Take your left index finger and place it in line with the middle of the nose and beneath your left eye.

-Once your left finger is in position, pull downwards very gently. Try to close your left eye in order to provide resistance against your finger.

-Hold the position as you count to five. Release and start again until you do the exercise ten times.

When you notice bags under your eyes, don't be quick to jump to conclusion that your lower eyelid is drooping especially if the bags seemingly appeared overnight. First, try to find out the cause before starting on the exercises.

Crow's Feet (eye exercise)

Your eyes perform very many functions among them helping you to see then sending signals to the brain and helping you judge situations. They also help you express your emotions. When you laugh, smile or even squint, wrinkles tend to form around your eyes. Small fold lines appear resembling the feet of crows, hence the name crow's feet. As you continue to grow older and continue to express your emotions, these folds take on a permanent shape. This is especially visible in elderly people, as they have accumulated a lot folds over the years. You can however use face yoga to eliminate wrinkles or greatly reduce their appearance. In order to get rid of crow's feet, you should:

-Take your right index finger and place it at the side of your right eye in a vertical position.

-Take your left index finger and place it at the side of your left eye in a vertical position. Ensure that you do not poke your eyes, as this will lead to unnecessary pain.

-Hold your fingers in place to prevent movement. Then slowly close your eyes. You will find that your fingers provide resistance such that when you close your eyes, you will feel as if you are pulling at them.

-Close your eyes for a moment and then open them. Keep repeating this exercise up to twenty times. Opening and closing your eyes.

-If you need more resistance than your fingers are offering, consider putting your fingers just at the inside corners of your eyes. This should done lightly and you should always ensure that your fingers are very clean. Your eyes are quite sensitive. You do not want to solve one problem only to end up with a bigger one. Be gentle when exercising your eyes. After you are done with your eyes, you can proceed to get rid of the nasal labial folds.

Nasal Labial Folds

When you laugh, folds appear above your mouth (on both sides) and along your nose. These folds are usually referred to as laugh lines. However, there is nothing funny about the folds when they take up permanent residency on your face even if you are not laughing. The folds make your cheeks sag, and make you look old and tired. Facial exercises will help you to eliminate the nasal labial folds and tighten your cheek muscles. In order to exercise your nasal labial folds, you should:

-Find a chair and sit down with your back touching the chair.

-Say 'aah', not literally but you get the point. Separate your upper teeth from the lower teeth – the further the better.

-Slowly move your head back such that your eyes will eventually look at the ceiling or the sky if you are outside.

-Stay that way for fifteen to twenty seconds without moving. This should give the muscles a good work out.

However, you can skip that step and head right to the 'puppet face' exercise (more like clown face actually). For this exercise, you should:

-Smile wide enough such that your face looks like the picture of a laughing clown. Ensure that your teeth are showing. Your upper teeth should not touch your lower teeth.

-As you smile, you will notice the folds near your mouth (in between your mouth and your nose on both sides of your face). Take four fingers of your right hand and place them on the folds of your right side. Then take four fingers of your left hand and place them on the folds of your left creases.

-After your fingers are in place, use them to provide resistance as you lift the muscles up. Hold for a while before releasing.

-As you continue doing the facial exercises, you should be able to notice some improvement on your face as your cheeks become firmer. While these exercise is good, taking care of the nasal labial folds is only one part of the equation. You need to exercise your cheeks to enjoy greater benefits.

Cheek Exercise

Your cheeks occupy a large part of your face. But, more than that, they contribute a big deal to your facial expressions. You can tell when someone is happy or sad just from the way their cheeks are placed on their face. Round cheeks often signify health and youth whereas hollow cheeks make one seem old and tired. This is why many people turn to Botox – because they want to keep their cheeks looking good.

As you get older, your cheeks begin to sag as they lose their elasticity. Not only do the cheeks sag but they also contribute to the sagging of your mouth corners, giving you a sad-faced look even when you are far from sad. In order to prevent this, you need to exercise your cheek muscles to make them firm. You should:

-Breathe in air through your mouth.

-After you take in air, puff out your cheeks until they resemble an air filled balloon.

-Do not release the air out. Instead, count up to five before letting it out. Repeat the exercise several times.

This exercise is intended to exercise the whole of your cheek. But, there are specific exercises for the upper cheek and the middle cheek. In order to exercise the upper part of your cheek, you should:

-Take your right hand fingers and place them on top of your right cheek in a horizontal position below your eye. Then take your left hand fingers and place them horizontally on top of your left cheek below your eye.

-After your fingers are firmly in place, smile. This way, your fingers will provide resistance as your corners of your mouth and your cheeks start moving upwards. Your fingers, in this instance, will act as weights. This will give the needed toning exercise to your upper cheeks.

-After smiling and lifting your cheeks upwards, count to five before returning your mouth to a neutral position. You should do this at least fifteen to twenty times.

Once you are finished with the upper part of your cheeks, it is time to exercise the middle part of your cheek. In this exercise, your aim will be to use your fingers as weights in order to firm your cheek muscles. In order to do this, you should:

-Take your right index finger and place it on the middle of the right cheek in a horizontal position. It should be at par with your nostrils. Then take your left index finger and place it on the middles of your left cheek in a horizontal position.

-Once both your fingers are in place, you should form your lips into a smile. As you do this, you should feel as if your cheeks are lifting your fingers. If you don't feel this, adjust your fingers accordingly.

-After you use your cheeks to lift your fingers, hold the position and count up to five before relaxing. You should repeat this exercise fifteen to twenty times.

These cheek exercises will contribute to the firming of your cheeks and give your cheeks that healthy and youthful look.

Mouth Exercise

When your mouth loses its elasticity, your face tends to acquire a sad appearance as the skin sags downwards. Exercising the muscles will lead to your mouth acquiring a youthful look. Your lips will also benefit from the exercises. In order to exercise your mouth, you should:

Take your right index finger and place it inside the corner of your right side of the mouth. Then take your left index finger and place it inside the left corner of your left side of your mouth. Let your fingers follow the shape of your mouth instead of hanging on nothing.

-Once your fingers are in place, begin pulling your mouth closed to the right and left simultaneously. Endeavor to make an 'o' shape with your mouth. The pull from your fingers will work to resist the forming of the shape.

-Hold the position before relaxing. Repeat the exercise up to forty times before stopping.

The corners of your mouth tend to sag over time especially if your cheeks droop. In order to exercise the corners of your mouth, you should:

-Take your right index finger and place it inside your mouth while placing your right thumb on the outside area such that you have a good hold on the skin.

-Take your left index finger and place it inside your left corner of the mouth while placing your left thumb on the outside ensuring you have a good grip.

-Try bringing the corners of your mouth together the way you would do when you want to whistle a tune. Your fingers should serve as resistance to make the muscles tone up.

-Hold for a moment before relaxing. Repeat this exercise up to thirty times.

The muscles around your mouth also need to be exercised. In order to do this, you should:

-Purse your lips. Your lips should feel as if they are pressing on each other.

-Take your right index finger and place it on the right corner of your mouth.

-Take your left index finger and place it on the left corner of your mouth.

-After your fingers are in place, start making circular motions with your fingers. This motion should be used to push the corners of your mouth up and down.

-Repeat the motion, counting up to thirty. Keep your lips pressed together tightly and don't fret when you feel a burning sensation.

Once you are done with your mouth exercises, you can now concentrate on improving the appearance of your lips.

Lips Exercise

Your lips play many roles. They enable you to retain fluids and solids inside your mouth. They also act as protection from undesirable objects entering your mouth. They allow you to articulate as you form words, and they also allow you to show facial expressions as well as kiss. Thus, it is vital that you take care of your lips. Unfortunately, since your lips do not possess sweat glands, they tend to dry up and become chapped. As you grow older, your lips start thinning. Having thin, dry, and chapped lips is not desirable at all. Fortunately, face yoga can help you have fuller lips. In order to exercise your lips, you should:

-Take a gulp of air. Ensure that your cheeks are only half full of air before you start to shift the air inside your mouth from the right cheek to the left cheek. This action is targeted at the tiny lines that surround your mouth. Move the air up to five times on each side of your mouth.

-Put your lips in a kissing position. You can make a kissing sound if this will help you. Kissing utilizes four muscles and thus helps exercise your lips muscles. Hold your lips in the kissing position before relaxing them. You should do this exercise up to thirty times.

-Make a fish face with your cheeks sucked inside your mouth. Hold this position and count up to five before releasing. Repeat this exercise up to twenty times.

-The next exercise requires you to open your mouth widely. Ensure that you feel your mouth stretching and then hold the position to the count of ten before relaxing. Do this up to five times.

-Press your lips inwards against each other. Pop your lips making the popping sound. Repeat the exercise up to ten times.

-Your lips tend to dry up quickly because they do not have their own moisture. It is therefore advisable that you moisturize your lips before engaging in any lip exercise. You should also drink water to keep yourself hydrated.

Jowls

Many people find it difficult to exercise their jowls simply because the jowls' muscles are ill developed. As you start exercising them, you may be unsure as to the effect. This is because you may not feel the effect of the exercise as you are doing it. However, when the skin on your jaw starts to sag, it does not present a beautiful sight. This area needs to be exercised and with time, you will start to feel its effects. In order to exercise the jowls muscles, you should:

-Lift your right hand to your right side of your jaw line and place four fingers horizontally such that the little finger sits at the end of your mouth. Do the same to your left side by placing your fingers on your left side of the jaw line.

-Once your hands are in place, smile. This action will enable you to move your mouth corners in an upward direction. At this point, you may feel a slight movement as the muscle moves your fingers. You should repeat this exercise at least twenty times.

You may also engage in a more noticeable exercise once you finish exercising your jowls muscle. In order to do this, you should:

-Begin by opening your mouth wide. Your jaw will move downwards.

-Once your mouth is open, proceed to push your jaw forward. This action will result in a pulling feeling especially in your cheeks. You should hold the position for at least ten seconds.

-Afterwards, push your jaw inwards. You may need to press your lips inwards for this to work. Proceed to hold the position for ten seconds before returning your jaw to a neutral position. You should do this exercise up to ten times.

Over time, you will begin to notice significant change as your jowls become tighter. So keep up with your jowls exercise.

Chin Exercise

When skin sagging is combined with fat accumulation, the result makes it look like an individual has a double chin – a situation often associated with someone being overweight (even when he or she is not). In order to eliminate this situation, you need to tone your chin and your jaw. You should:

-Find a comfortable chair, preferably one with a straight back rest, to sit on. Then proceed to look up to the ceiling such that your chin is facing upwards.

-Once your chin is pointing upwards, proceed to push your jaw in front without opening your mouth.

-Count up to ten, then lower your chin to a neutral position with your eyes looking straight ahead.

-Repeat the exercise up to twenty times before stopping.

-As you exercise your chin to get rid of the double chin, ensure that you also work on eating a healthy diet so that you can also get rid of excessive fat.

Neck Exercise

When the skin on your neckline sags, you end up with a 'turkey neck' and if you have ever seen turkeys, you would know that this is definitely not a compliment. In order to get rid of the turkey neck, you should:

-Sit down on a chair and open your mouth. You should try to put as much space as possible between your lower teeth and your upper teeth.

-As you open your mouth, try pulling your mouth corners towards your neck without using your hands. The goal is to strengthen your neck muscles.

-Hold this position for five seconds before relaxing. You should repeat this exercise at least ten times.

Another area, of concern is developing a double chin. This situation affects both the chin and the neck muscles. In order to get rid of the undesirable double chin, you should:

-Tilt your neck backwards as far as you can without hurting yourself.

-Touch the roof of your mouth with your tongue and hold that position for at least ten seconds before relaxing.

-Be careful when doing neck exercises as you do not want to injure your throat muscles while engaging in face yoga.

Lion Face Exercise

Once you have engaged in the various facial exercises, it is time to give your face one final workout. You can do this by engaging in an exercise known as lion face due to the resemblance of the face of a lion when doing it. In order to do this exercise, you should:

-Kneel down on the floor, preferably on a mat to protect your knees. You can sit on the heels of your legs.

-Take in a deep breath. Bend your hands at the elbows in a vertical position and form a fist with both hands.

-When your hands are in place, proceed to squeeze your face muscles so that they resemble the face a child makes when they are frightened and closing their eyes to avoid seeing something bad. Ensure that you squeeze hard. You may feel discomfort as you do this especially in your eyes.

-Breathe out through your mouth. Open your mouth and stick your tongue out as far as you can.

-Proceed to open your eyes wide and then roll them several times then let your palm open, stretching your fingers wide. You should do this exercise at least two times.

Once you are done with the lion face, your face yoga session is practically over. However, just like any other exercise, you need to ease out of the exercise routine.

Wrapping up after Facial Exercises

This is the final stage. It comes after the lion face stage. This is the stage where you reset your face as it were. It is sometimes called Buddha face because of the tranquility it projects. Your face should be in a neutral position i.e. without facial expressions. The only thing you should do is have a gentle smile on your face.

Conclusion

Face yoga is good for your face. It helps you tone your facial muscles, remove wrinkles, and makes you look younger. However, it cannot be done in isolation. Keep in mind that your face needs protection from the sun and harsh elements. It also needs cleansing due to the dirt particles and other pathogens in the air. In order to reap the best results, combine diet, personal care and skin protection with your face yoga routine. Do not give up on the way. It takes time to exercise muscles but you will begin seeing favorable results. Study the facial exercises from time to time and embark on doing them routinely to get rid of wrinkles and enjoy a younger looking face.

Bonus Content!

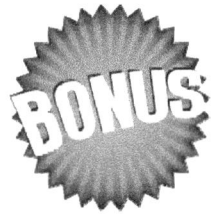

As a token of our appreciation Grand Reveur Publications would like to give you access to our exclusive bonus content (including free eBooks!).

You're only a click away from receiving:

Exclusive pre-release access to our latest eBooks

Free Grand Reveur eBooks during promotional periods

A method ANYONE can use to publish their own book and make passive income

https://ignorelimits.leadpages.net/grandreveur publications/

As this is a limited time offer it would be a shame to miss out, I recommend grabbing these bonuses before reading on.